Series MB3 no.19

Congenital Anomaly Statistics Notifications

A statistical review of notifications of congenital anomalies received as part of the England and Wales National Congenital Anomaly System, 2004

METROPOLITAN BOROUGH OF WIRRAL

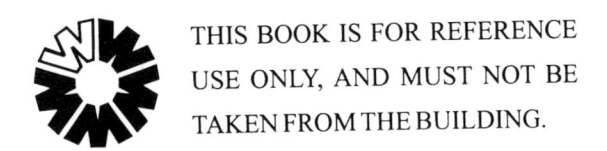

THIS BOOK IS FOR REFERENCE USE ONLY, AND MUST NOT BE TAKEN FROM THE BUILDING.

EDUCATION & CULTURAL SERVICES DEPARTMENT

© Crown copyright 2005
Published with the permission of the Controller of Her Majesty's
Stationery Office (HMSO)

ISBN **1 857774 615 5**
ISSN **1460-3934**

This publication, excluding logos, may be reproduced free of charge, in any format or medium for research or private study subject to it being reproduced accurately and not used in a misleading context. The material must be acknowledged as crown copyright and the title of the publication specified. This publication can also be accessed at the National Statistics website: **www.statistics.gov.uk**

For any other use of this material please apply for a free Click-Use Licence on the Office of Public Sector Information (OPSI) website:
www.opsi.gov.uk/click-use/index.htm
Or write to The Licensing Division, St Clement's House, 2-16 Colegate, Norwich NR3 1BQ. Fax 01603 723000 or e-mail: hmsolicensing@cabinetoffice.x.gsi.gov.uk

Contact points
For enquiries about this publication, contact
Denise Anderson
Tel: **01329 813204**
E-mail: **denise.anderson@ons.gov.uk**

For general enquiries, contact the National Statistics
Customer Contact Centre on: **0845 601 3034**
(minicom: 01633 812399)
E-mail: **info@statistics.gsi.gov.uk**
Fax: 01633 652747
Post: Room 1015, Government Buildings,
Cardiff Road, Newport NP10 8XG

You can also find National Statistics on the Internet at:
www.statistics.gov.uk

About the Office for National Statistics
The Office for National Statistics (ONS) is the government agency responsible for compiling, analysing and disseminating economic, social and demographic statistics about the United Kingdom. It also administers the statutory registration of births, marriages and deaths in England and Wales. The Director of ONS is also the National Statistician and the Registrar General for England and Wales.

A National Statistics publication
National Statistics are produced to high professional standards set out in the National Statistics Code of Practice. They are produced free from political influence.

Contents

			Page
Introduction			v
General notes			vii
Table 1	Summary table – Congenital anomaly notifications, Abortion notifications, 2004	England and Wales	1
Table 2a	Live and stillborn babies notified - numbers: sex by condition, 2004	England and Wales	2
Table 2b	Live and stillborn babies notified - rates per 10,000 live/stillbirths: sex by condition, 2004	England and Wales	3
Table 3	All babies notified - numbers: number of reported anomalies, 2004	England and Wales	4
Table 4a	Live and stillborn babies notified - numbers: multiplicity by condition, 2004	England and Wales	5
Table 4b	Live and stillborn babies notified - rates per 10,000 live/stillbirths: multiplicity by condition, 2004	England and Wales	5
Table 5a	Total (live and still) births, all babies notified - numbers: condition by area of usual residence of mother, 2004	England and Wales	6
Table 5b	All babies notified - rates per 10,000 total births: condition by area of usual residence of mother, 2004	England and Wales	8
Table 6a	All babies notified - numbers: month of birth by condition, 2004	England and Wales	10
Table 6b	All babies notified - rates per 10,000 total births: month of birth by condition, 2004	England and Wales	10
Table 7a	Live and stillborn babies notified - numbers: birthweight by condition, 2004	England and Wales	12
Table 7b	Live and stillborn babies notified - rates per 10,000 live/stillbirths: birthweight by condition, 2004	England and Wales	13
Table 8a	All babies notified - numbers: age of mother by condition, 2004	England and Wales	14
Table 8b	All babies notified - rates per 10,000 total births: age of mother by condition, 2004	England and Wales	14
Table 9	Strategic Health Authorities in England, and Wales which have shown an increase of numbers of a particular anomaly compared with the average notification for that area and anomaly during a previous period, 2004	England and Wales	15

			Page
Appendix A	List of conditions for exclusion		**16**
Appendix B	Example of congenital anomalies notifications form (SD56)		**17**
Appendix C	List of ICD10 codes included within anomaly groups		**18**
Appendix D	ONS Monitoring groups and ICD10 equivalent codes		**19**
Appendix E	Summary table - Congenital anomaly notifications, Abortion notifications, Stillbirths, Neonatal deaths, 2003	England and Wales	**21**

Introduction

The monitoring scheme

This is the nineteenth in a series of annual reference volumes and presents information collected through the National Congenital Anomaly System (NCAS) for 2004.[1]

Since 1964 the Office for National Statistics (ONS) has run a monitoring system for congenital anomalies in England and Wales. This notification system was initiated following the thalidomide epidemic in order to quickly detect any similar hazard. The primary purpose of this system is to detect changes in the frequency of reporting any particular anomaly or group of anomalies rather than trying to estimate the prevalence at birth. From 1st January 1995 anomalies detected at any age can be reported to the NCAS.

The congenital anomaly notification system, which is voluntary at all stages, is usually linked to the statutory system of birth notification to local health authorities which has existed since 1926. The local health authorities extract from the birth notifications details of babies born with anomalies. This information is commonly supplemented with details obtained from midwives, hospitals, doctors and health visitors.

Prior to 1990 all anomalies, however minor, were reportable to ONS. In January 1990 an exclusion list was introduced (a copy of the exclusion list is at **Appendix A**). This list describes the minor anomalies which should no longer be notified to ONS.

Information about babies with congenital anomalies is forwarded to ONS on a standard form (a copy of the reporting form used for the period covered by this volume is at **Appendix B**). Following the restructuring of the National Health Service in 1974 the information was passed to ONS by the area health authorities (AHAs) and their respective area Medical Officers. When AHAs were abolished in March 1982 the work was taken over by the district health authorities (DHAs) and their district Medical Officers.

Since the reforms following the NHS and Community Care Act 1990, the notification forms have been completed by NHS Trusts, which receive birth notifications on behalf of the Health Authority.

Significant changes have taken place in the organisation of the National Health Service in recent years. This volume relates to the situation as it existed in 2004.

ONS performs a statistical analysis on every quarter's notifications. This analysis uses the cumulative sum (CUSUM) technique. This compares the number of notifications in each of the nearly 100 anomalies or groups of anomalies (see **Appendix D**) in each of the areas monitored, with the average number previously reported from that area. If a significant rise is detected in any monitored class or group the relevant health authorities are informed. It must be remembered that an increase in notification may be due to changes in reporting practice rather than due to a true change in prevalence.

From the notification form at **Appendix B**, it can be seen that information is also collected on a number of factors of interest which are not apparently directly relevant to the monitoring, including parents' occupations and mother's age. These factors are used for epidemiological studies.

Although NCAS is primarily for monitoring changes in the frequency of reporting anomalies, it does provide the most extensive data on the prevalence levels available in England and Wales. However the major disadvantage of using the monitoring system to measure prevalence arises from the deficiencies in its coverage. In 1996 the Registrar General's Medical Advisory Committee[2] recommended that '*Where good congenital anomaly registers exist outside OPCS (now ONS) information should be exchanged with these registers*'.

Local congenital anomaly registers started exchanging data electronically with ONS in the year as listed below.

1998 - Welsh Congenital Anomaly Register and Information Service (CARIS)[3]
1999 - East Midlands & South Yorkshire Congenital Anomaly Register
2000 - North Thames (West) Congenital Malformation Register
 - Merseyside and Cheshire Congenital Anomaly Survey
2002 - Wessex Antenatally Detected Anomalies Register (WANDA)
 - Congenital Anomaly Register for Oxfordshire, Berkshire & Buckinghamshire (CAROBB) *(only covers Oxfordshire up to 2003)*
2003 - Northern Congenital Abnormality Register (NorCas)
 - South West Congenital Anomaly Register

In April 2001, a revised guide for data users and suppliers was distributed.[4] The purpose of this handbook was to provide information about the National System, guidance about reporting anomalies for data suppliers and information about surveillance for health authorities.

Symbols and conventions used

- nil
.. not available
* In line with the National Statistics Code of Practice and the underpinning Protocol on Data Access and Confidentiality, all statistics have been disclosure-controlled to protect confidentiality. Thus all subnational numbers smaller than 5 on live and stillborn babies have been suppressed. However, for abortion statistics less than 10 cases have been suppressed (See General notes - abortions, for more details). All rates based on such numbers have also been suppressed. Secondary suppressions have been applied as necessary to avoid the possibility of disclosure through subtraction.

Rates calculated from less than 20 anomalies are distinguished by italic type as a warning to the user that their reliability as a measure may be affected by the small number of events.

References

1. Annual update: Congenital anomaly statistics: notifications, 2004 England and Wales. *Health Statistics Quarterly* **29**. To be published February 2006.
2. The OPCS Monitoring Scheme for Congenital Malformations. A review of the Registrar General's Medical Advisory Committee. Occasional Paper 43 (1995) HMSO: London.
3. Botting B (2000). The impact of more complete data from Wales on the National Congenital Anomaly System. *Health Statistics Quarterly* **05**, 7-9.
4. Office for National Statistics (2001). *The National Congenital Anomaly System – A guide for data users and suppliers.*
www.statistics.gov.uk/statbase/Product.asp?vlnk=3115

General notes

The statistics in this publication relate to the National Congenital Anomaly System (NCAS) as at 1 September 2005.

All tables relate to 2004 data only: no time series data have been included.

Congenital Anomalies

Since 1995 congenital anomaly notifications have been classified to the *International Statistical Classification of Diseases and Related Health Problems* tenth Revision (ICD10). This allowed some conditions which had previously been within a single ICD9 code, to be identified separately, for example *gastroschisis* and *exomphalos* to be shown separately. Details of the ICD10 codes which are included in the major anomaly categories in the tables can be found in **Appendix C**.

Age at death

Stillbirths   late fetal deaths:
                   Until 30 September 1992:
                   after 28 weeks of gestation.
                   From 1 October 1992:
                   after 24 weeks of gestation.

Neonatal deaths   Deaths in the first 4 weeks of life
                   (ie 27 completed days)

Causes of death

Number of neonatal deaths and stillbirths in 2004 by selected congenital anomalies will be published in Spring 2006 in the ONS publication - Series DH3 Mortality statistics: childhood, infant and perinatal 2004. Figures for 2003 are shown in **Appendix E**.

Abortions

Number of abortions that are shown in **Table 1** have been compiled from notifications of abortions that are completed by the operating practitioners under the 1967 Abortion Act and are sent to the Chief Medical Officers of England and Wales. Section 37 of the Human Fertilisation and Embryology Act 1990 made changes to the Abortion Act 1967. These changes came into effect on 1 April 1991 and principally altered the statutory grounds under which abortions may be performed, and the time limit within which they may be carried out.

A legally induced abortion must be:

a) performed by a registered medical practitioner,
b) performed except in an emergency, in a National Health Service hospital or in a place approved for the purpose of the Act, and
c) certified by two registered medical practitioners as necessary on any of the grounds:

A the continuance of the pregnancy would involve a risk to the life of the pregnant woman greater than if the pregnancy was terminated;

B the termination is necessary to prevent grave permanent injury to the health of the pregnant woman;

C the continuance of the pregnancy would involve risk greater than if the pregnancy were terminated, of injury to the physical or mental health of the pregnant woman;

D the continuance of the pregnancy would involve risk greater than if the pregnancy were terminated to the physical or mental health of any existing child(ren) of the family of the pregnant woman;

E there is a substantial risk that if the child were born it would suffer from such physical or mental abnormalities as to be seriously handicapped;

or in an emergency, certified by the operating practitioner as immediately necessary

F to save the life of the pregnant woman;

or

G to prevent grave permanent injury to the physical or mental health of the woman.

The abortion notifications reported in this volume are those carried out under grounds E either alone or in combination with grounds A, B, C or D. The notification form required information about the medical condition found or reported and any diagnosis or suspected condition of the fetus. The medical conditions have been classified to ICD10.

Recommendations from the National Statistics Disclosure Review

Since April 2002, the Department of Health has been responsible for the processing of the abortions notification forms and information has been made accessible to the Office for National Statistics (ONS) for statistical purposes.

In releasing health statistics, usually with small numbers, there is a risk that it may lead to identifying individuals. To address this, the Department of Health asked the National Statistician to provide guidelines for interpreting the National Statistics Code of Practice and assorted protocols when handling health statistics, in a way that balances data confidentiality risks with the public interest in the use of these figures. In July 2005, ONS published a report on disclosure guidance for abortion statistics. This can be found on the ONS website at:

www.statistics.gov.uk/statbase/Product.asp?vlnk=11988

As recommended by the review, abortion data in **Table 1** and **Appendix E** are suppressed for conditions where there were fewer than 10 cases (ie 0–9 cases).

Area of residence

Tables 5a and **5b** show data by Government Office Region and Strategic Health Authority of residence of mother at the time of the child's birth.

Birthweight

ONS has obtained birthweight for live births since 1975 through the co-operation of district health authorities. Birthweight information given on the birth notification form is transferred from district health authorities to the local registrars of births and deaths who copy it on to the birth registration draft entry forms. These are subsequently forwarded to ONS for statistical processing. A similar system operates for stillbirths, although the initial source of information is the medical certificate which is prepared by the certifying doctor or midwife, and is passed, usually by the parent, to the registrar.

In 2004, 99.8 per cent of live births and 97.5 per cent of stillbirths had a birthweight recorded.

Further information

ONS is happy to provide statistics to outside researchers pursuing related topics subject to the constraints of confidentiality. Particulars relating to individual (anonymous) children are only released with the approval of the data custodian (usually a community paediatrician within the Community Trust), who originally provided the data. Anyone interested in using these data should contact:

Child Health Unit
Office for National Statistics
Room B6/10
1 Drummond Gate
London SW1V 2QQ
Telephone: 020 7533 5641 or
ncas@ons.gov.uk

Series MB3 no.19 Table 1 2004

Table 1 Summary table showing congenital anomaly statistics from two systems **England and Wales**
National Congenital Anomaly System, Abortion Statistics, 2004

Condition	Congenital anomaly notifications (NCAS)[1]			Abortion notifications (under grounds E)[2]
	Live birth	Stillbirth	Not known	
All babies notified	**6,023**	**322**	**13**	**1,894**
Babies with a mention of:				
Central nervous system anomalies	277	82	3	443
Anencephalus	12	10	-	145
All spina bifida	58	17	3	90
Encephalocele	12	2	-	19
Congenital hydrocephalus	52	20	-	52
Eye	99	3	1	*
Anophthalmia	7	2	-	*
Cleft lip and palate	483	16	1	*
Cleft of only lip	123	3	-	*
Cleft of only palate	157	7	-	*
Cleft of lip and palate	203	6	1	*
Other face, ear and neck	151	7	1	*
Heart and circulatory	1,158	74	2	147
Respiratory	131	15	-	28
Alimentary	390	25	1	*
Tracheo-oesophageal fistula	48	2	-	*
Oesophageal atresia	13	2	-	*
Atresia/stenosis large intestine, rectum or anal canal	78	3	-	*
Genital organs	515	6	-	*
Hypospadias	410	1	-	*
Urinary system	694	29	2	69
Renal agenesis/dysgenesis	61	8	-	24
Epispadias	12	-	-	*
Musculoskeletal	1,855	69	2	124
Dislocation of hip	103	1	-	*
Deformities of feet	530	18	-	*
Polydactyly	307	4	-	*
Syndactyly	159	3	-	*
Limb reductions	187	8	1	*
Diaphragmatic defects	77	10	-	18
Exomphalos	50	7	-	11
Gastroschisis	186	5	-	*
Skin and integument	213	5	2	*
Chromosomal anomalies	596	81	4	726
Down syndrome	420	34	2	419
Endocrine and metabolic disorders	150	3	-	*
Congenital infections	9	2	-	..
Other congenital anomalies not elsewhere classified	382	57	2	56

Note: For more information on stillbirths, neonatal deaths and abortions data: see page vii.
Source
1 National Congenital Anomaly System at 1st September 2005.
2 Department of Health. Abortion Statistics, England and Wales 2004, July 2005.

* less than 10 cases

Table 2a 2004 Series MB3 no.19

Table 2a Live and stillborn babies notified - numbers: sex by condition, 2004

England and Wales

Condition	Total[1] Total[2]	Male	Female	Live born Total[2]	Male	Female	Stillborn Total[2]	Male	Female
All babies notified	**6,358**	**3,661**	**2,648**	**6,023**	**3,493**	**2,501**	**322**	**163**	**141**
Babies with a mention of:									
Central nervous system anomalies	**362**	189	164	277	148	126	82	41	35
Anencephalus	**22**	9	10	12	6	6	10	3	4
All spina bifida	**78**	35	41	58	29	28	17	6	10
Encephalocele	**14**	8	6	12	7	5	2	1	1
Congenital hydrocephalus	**72**	45	26	52	34	17	20	11	9
Eye	**103**	50	53	99	48	51	3	1	2
Anophthalmia	**9**	5	4	7	4	3	2	1	1
Cleft lip and palate	**500**	290	206	483	285	196	16	4	10
Cleft of only lip	**126**	82	43	123	81	41	3	1	2
Cleft of only palate	**164**	67	96	157	67	90	7	-	6
Cleft of lip and palate	**210**	141	67	203	137	65	6	3	2
Other face, ear and neck	**159**	74	83	151	71	78	7	3	4
Heart and circulatory	**1,234**	632	595	1,158	592	562	74	40	33
Respiratory	**146**	70	75	131	64	66	15	6	9
Alimentary	**416**	250	163	390	232	155	25	18	7
Tracheo-oesophageal fistula	**50**	30	20	48	28	20	2	2	-
Oesophageal atresia	**15**	9	6	13	8	5	2	1	1
Atresia/stenosis large intestine, rectum or anal canal	**81**	48	31	78	46	30	3	2	1
Genital organs	**521**	458	48	515	455	48	6	3	-
Hypospadias	**411**	408	2	410	407	2	1	1	-
Urinary system	**725**	485	232	694	470	219	29	14	13
Renal agenesis/dysgenesis	**69**	39	29	61	34	26	8	5	3
Epispadias	**12**	12	-	12	12	-	-	-	-
Musculoskeletal	**1,926**	1,031	889	1,855	993	857	69	38	30
Dislocation of the hip	**104**	24	80	103	24	79	1	-	1
Deformities of feet	**548**	301	246	530	289	240	18	12	6
Polydactyly	**311**	185	126	307	184	123	4	1	3
Syndactyly	**162**	108	54	159	106	53	3	2	1
Limb reductions	**196**	103	93	187	98	89	8	5	3
Diaphragmatic defects	**87**	48	38	77	44	32	10	4	6
Exomphalos	**57**	33	24	50	28	22	7	5	2
Gastroschisis	**191**	100	89	186	97	87	5	3	2
Skin and integument	**220**	107	113	213	101	112	5	4	1
Chromosomal anomalies	**681**	353	323	596	313	281	81	38	41
Down syndrome	**456**	245	209	420	224	194	34	20	14
Endocrine and metabolic disorders	**153**	77	76	150	75	75	3	2	1
Congenital infections	**11**	7	3	9	7	2	2	-	1
Other congenital anomalies not elsewhere classified	**441**	242	193	382	211	170	57	29	23
Total live and stillbirths	**643,026**	**330,086**	**312,940**	**639,509**	**328,227**	**311,282**	**3,517**	**1,859**	**1,658**

1 Total includes unknown whether live or stillborn.
2 Includes indeterminate sex and not known/not stated.

Table 2b Live and stillborn babies notified - rates per 10,000 live/stillbirths: sex by condition, 2004 — England and Wales

Condition	Live born Male	Live born Female	Stillborn Male	Stillborn Female
All babies notified	**106.4**	**80.3**	**876.8**	**850.4**
Babies with a mention of:				
Central nervous system anomalies	4.5	4.0	220.5	211.1
Anencephalus	0.2	0.2	16.1	24.1
All spina bifida	0.9	0.9	32.3	60.3
Encephalocele	0.2	0.2	5.4	6.0
Congenital hydrocephalus	1.0	0.5	59.2	54.3
Eye	1.5	1.6	5.4	12.1
Anophthalmia	0.1	0.1	5.4	6.0
Cleft lip and palate	8.7	6.3	21.5	60.3
Cleft of only lip	2.5	1.3	5.4	12.1
Cleft of only palate	2.0	2.9	-	36.2
Cleft of lip and palate	4.2	2.1	16.1	12.1
Other face, ear and neck	2.2	2.5	16.1	24.1
Heart and circulatory	18.0	18.1	215.2	199.0
Respiratory	1.9	2.1	32.3	54.3
Alimentary	7.1	5.0	96.8	42.2
Tracheo-oesophageal fistula	0.9	0.6	10.8	-
Oesophageal atresia	0.2	0.2	5.4	6.0
Atresia/stenosis large intestine, rectum or anal canal	1.4	1.0	10.8	6.0
Genital organs	13.9	1.5	16.1	-
Hypospadias	12.4	0.1	5.4	-
Urinary system	14.3	7.0	75.3	78.4
Renal agenesis/dysgenesis	1.0	0.8	26.9	18.1
Epispadias	0.4	-	-	-
Musculoskeletal	30.3	27.5	204.4	180.9
Dislocation of the hip	0.7	2.5	-	6.0
Deformities of feet	8.8	7.7	64.6	36.2
Polydactyly	5.6	4.0	5.4	18.1
Syndactyly	3.2	1.7	10.8	6.0
Limb reductions	3.0	2.9	26.9	18.1
Diaphragmatic defects	1.3	1.0	21.5	36.2
Exomphalos	0.9	0.7	26.9	12.1
Gastroschisis	3.0	2.8	16.1	12.1
Skin and integument	3.1	3.6	21.5	6.0
Chromosomal anomalies	9.5	9.0	204.4	247.3
Down syndrome	6.8	6.2	107.6	84.4
Endocrine and metabolic disorders	2.3	2.4	10.8	6.0
Congenital infections	0.2	0.1	-	6.0
Other congenital anomalies not elsewhere classified	6.4	5.5	156.0	138.7

Table 3   All babies notified - numbers: **England and Wales**
          number of reported anomalies, 2004

All babies notified	6,358
1 anomaly	4,875
2 anomalies	935
3 anomalies	311
4 anomalies	136
5 anomalies	50
6 anomalies	28
7 anomalies	14
8 or more anomalies	9

Series MB3 no.19 Tables 4a and 4b 2004

Table 4a Live and stillborn babies notified - numbers: multiplicity by condition, 2004 England and Wales

Condition	Total[1]			Live born			Stillborn		
	Total[2]	Singleton	Multiple	Total[2]	Singleton	Multiple	Total[2]	Singleton	Multiple
All babies notified	6,358	6,095	221	6,023	5,796	186	322	288	34
Babies with a mention of:									
Central nervous system anomalies	362	332	29	277	263	13	82	66	16
Anencephalus	22	14	8	12	8	4	10	6	4
All spina bifida	78	72	6	58	57	1	17	12	5
Eye	103	98	3	99	95	3	3	3	-
Cleft lip and palate	500	478	11	483	463	9	16	14	2
Other face, ear and neck	159	153	5	151	146	4	7	6	1
Heart and circulatory	1,234	1,164	56	1,158	1,094	50	74	69	5
Respiratory	146	140	6	131	126	5	15	14	1
Alimentary	416	403	11	390	377	11	25	25	-
Genital organs	521	511	10	515	505	10	6	6	-
Urinary system	725	698	26	694	669	24	29	27	2
Musculoskeletal	1,926	1,865	58	1,855	1,799	53	69	64	5
Skin and integument	220	212	6	213	205	6	5	5	-
Chromosomal anomalies	681	653	20	596	573	15	81	76	5
Down syndrome	456	440	12	420	406	10	34	32	2
Endocrine and metabolic disorders	153	145	5	150	142	5	3	3	-
Congenital infections	11	11	-	9	9	-	2	2	-
Other congenital anomalies not elsewhere classified	441	417	20	382	365	13	57	50	7
Total live and stillbirths	643,026	623,992	19,034	639,509	620,741	18,768	3,517	3,251	266

1 Total includes unknown whether live or stillborn.
2 Includes not known/not stated.

Table 4b Live and stillborn babies notified - rates per 10,000 live/stillbirths: multiplicity by condition, 2004 England and Wales

Condition	Total[1]			Live born			Stillborn		
	Total[2]	Singleton	Multiple	Total[2]	Singleton	Multiple	Total[2]	Singleton	Multiple
All babies notified	98.9	97.7	116.1	94.2	93.4	99.1	915.6	885.9	1,278.2
Babies with a mention of:									
Central nervous system anomalies	5.6	5.3	15.2	4.3	4.2	6.9	233.2	203.0	601.5
Anencephalus	0.3	0.2	4.2	0.2	0.1	2.1	28.4	18.5	150.4
All spina bifida	1.2	1.2	3.2	0.9	0.9	0.5	48.3	36.9	188.0
Eye	1.6	1.6	1.6	1.5	1.5	1.6	8.5	9.2	-
Cleft lip and palate	7.8	7.7	5.8	7.6	7.5	4.8	45.5	43.1	75.2
Other face, ear and neck	2.5	2.5	2.6	2.4	2.4	2.1	19.9	18.5	37.6
Heart and circulatory	19.2	18.7	29.4	18.1	17.6	26.6	210.4	212.2	188.0
Respiratory	2.3	2.2	3.2	2.0	2.0	2.7	42.7	43.1	37.6
Alimentary	6.5	6.5	5.8	6.1	6.1	5.9	71.1	76.9	-
Genital organs	8.1	8.2	5.3	8.1	8.1	5.3	17.1	18.5	-
Urinary system	11.3	11.2	13.7	10.9	10.8	12.8	82.5	83.1	75.2
Musculoskeletal	30.0	29.9	30.5	29.0	29.0	28.2	196.2	196.9	188.0
Skin and integument	3.4	3.4	3.2	3.3	3.3	3.2	14.2	15.4	-
Chromosomal anomalies	10.6	10.5	10.5	9.3	9.2	8.0	230.3	233.8	188.0
Down syndrome	7.1	7.1	6.3	6.6	6.5	5.3	96.7	98.4	75.2
Endocrine and metabolic disorders	2.4	2.3	2.6	2.3	2.3	2.7	8.5	9.2	-
Congenital infections	0.2	0.2	-	0.1	0.1	-	5.7	6.2	-
Other congenital anomalies not elsewhere classified	6.9	6.7	10.5	6.0	5.9	6.9	162.1	153.8	263.2

1 Total includes unknown whether live or stillborn.
2 Includes not known/not stated.

Table 5a 2004 Series MB3 no.19

Table 5a Total (live and still) births, all babies notified - numbers:
condition by area of usual residence of mother, 2004

Area of usual residence	Total (live and still) births	Central nervous system anomalies	Cleft lip and palate	Other face, ear and neck	Heart and circulatory	Alimentary
ENGLAND AND WALES	**643,026**	**362**	**500**	**159**	**1,234**	**416**
England	**610,522**	**334**	**462**	**138**	**927**	**367**
Wales	**32,504**	**28**	**38**	**21**	**307**	**49**
Government Office Regions						
North East	27,972	21	32	*	210	16
North West	81,613	43	64	12	87	39
Yorkshire and The Humber	60,540	32	48	8	114	44
East Midlands	48,510	51	50	14	87	65
West Midlands	66,278	15	45	*	21	18
East	64,589	26	51	15	53	27
London	114,389	65	45	19	110	31
South East	94,092	49	78	24	94	48
South West	52,539	32	49	38	151	79
Strategic Health Authorities/ Government Regions						
North East						
County Durham and Tees Valley	13,223	11	17	*	72	7
Northumberland, Tyne and Wear	14,749	10	15	*	138	9
North West						
Cheshire and Merseyside	26,459	27	20	*	38	13
Cumbria and Lancashire	21,936	*	22	*	29	16
Greater Manchester	33,218	*	22	*	20	10
Yorkshire and The Humber						
North and East Yorkshire and Northern Lincolnshire	17,588	8	10	5	*	*
South Yorkshire	15,113	18	28	*	94	30
West Yorkshire	27,839	6	10	*	*	*
East Midlands						
Leicestershire, Northamptonshire and Rutland	19,522	27	17	6	42	29
Trent	28,988	24	33	8	44	36
West Midlands						
Birmingham and the Black Country	32,036	11	16	*	5	*
Shropshire and Staffordshire	16,739	*	21	*	11	9
West Midlands South	17,503	*	8	*	5	*
East						
Bedfordshire and Hertfordshire	21,032	15	24	*	27	*
Essex	19,000	*	10	6	7	*
Norfolk, Suffolk and Cambridgeshire	24,557	*	17	*	19	12
London						
North Central London	18,554	12	6	*	*	*
North East London	26,608	13	*	*	13	*
North West London	26,805	29	23	8	69	17
South East London	23,441	*	*	*	*	*
South West London	18,981	*	10	*	19	6
South East						
Hampshire and Isle of Wight	19,876	22	31	8	45	21
Kent and Medway	18,510	*	8	*	*	5
Surrey and Sussex	28,347	*	16	*	*	10
Thames Valley	27,359	20	23	12	36	12
South West						
Avon, Gloucestershire and Wiltshire	25,241	10	27	*	46	29
Dorset and Somerset	11,699	6	7	*	23	18
South West Peninsula	15,599	16	15	18	82	32

Series MB3 no.19 Table 5a 2004

England and Wales

Area of usual residence

Genital organs	Urinary system	Musculoskeletal	Skin and integument	Chromosomal anomalies	Down syndrome	Other congenital anomalies not elsewhere classified	
521	725	1,926	220	681	456	441	**ENGLAND AND WALES**
473	644	1,709	199	611	419	378	**England**
48	81	217	21	70	37	63	**Wales**
							Government Office Regions
13	46	75	7	75	50	15	North East
79	150	255	45	80	55	62	North West
59	36	135	6	43	31	21	Yorkshire and The Humber
94	91	280	8	89	65	41	East Midlands
33	43	124	12	23	17	31	West Midlands
39	44	117	25	56	45	44	East
41	73	219	54	81	52	66	London
53	65	207	17	95	66	58	South East
62	96	297	25	69	38	40	South West
							Strategic Health Authorities/ Government Regions
							North East
7	20	31	*	40	28	6	County Durham and Tees Valley
6	26	44	*	35	22	9	Northumberland, Tyne and Wear
							North West
26	104	103	8	36	25	18	Cheshire and Merseyside
22	14	58	21	20	14	30	Cumbria and Lancashire
31	32	94	16	24	16	14	Greater Manchester
							Yorkshire and The Humber
							North and East Yorkshire
10	*	40	*	*	*	*	and Northern Lincolnshire
43	29	66	*	22	16	12	South Yorkshire
6	*	29	*	*	*	*	West Yorkshire
							East Midlands
							Leicestershire, Northamptonshire
31	57	114	*	40	32	21	and Rutland
63	34	166	*	49	33	20	Trent
							West Midlands
23	37	62	8	8	6	25	Birmingham and the Black Country
*	*	26	*	8	6	*	Shropshire and Staffordshire
*	*	36	*	7	5	*	West Midlands South
							East
10	26	37	7	31	24	10	Bedfordshire and Hertfordshire
20	6	52	12	6	5	27	Essex
9	12	28	6	19	16	7	Norfolk, Suffolk and Cambridgeshire
							London
8	12	31	7	10	7	8	North Central London
11	*	63	*	*	*	7	North East London
14	32	75	10	53	31	27	North West London
*	*	22	28	*	*	15	South East London
*	16	28	*	8	6	9	South West London
							South East
7	19	61	*	41	26	20	Hampshire and Isle of Wight
9	10	30	*	6	5	5	Kent and Medway
18	17	34	5	13	11	9	Surrey and Sussex
19	19	82	9	35	24	24	Thames Valley
							South West
31	41	123	15	40	19	15	Avon, Gloucestershire and Wiltshire
10	17	38	*	16	10	11	Dorset and Somerset
21	38	136	*	13	9	14	South West Peninsula

Table 5b All babies notified - rates per 10,000 total births: condition by area of usual residence of mother, 2004

Area of usual residence

	Central nervous system anomalies	Cleft lip and palate	Other face, ear and neck	Heart and circulatory	Alimentary	Genital organs
ENGLAND AND WALES	**5.6**	**7.8**	**2.5**	**19.2**	**6.5**	**8.1**
England	**5.5**	**7.6**	**2.3**	**15.2**	**6.0**	**7.7**
Wales	**8.6**	**11.7**	**6.5**	**94.4**	**15.1**	**14.8**
Government Office Regions						
North East	7.5	11.4	*	75.1	5.7	4.6
North West	5.3	7.8	1.5	10.7	4.8	9.7
Yorkshire and The Humber	5.3	7.9	1.3	18.8	7.3	9.7
East Midlands	10.5	10.3	2.9	17.9	13.4	19.4
West Midlands	2.3	6.8	*	3.2	2.7	5.0
East	4.0	7.9	2.3	8.2	4.2	6.0
London	5.7	3.9	1.7	9.6	2.7	3.6
South East	5.2	8.3	2.6	10.0	5.1	5.6
South West	6.1	9.3	7.2	28.7	15.0	11.8

Series MB3 no.19 Table 5b 2004

England and Wales

Area of usual residence

Urinary system	Musculoskeletal	Skin and integument	Chromosomal anomalies	Down syndrome	Other congenital anomalies not elsewhere classified	
11.3	**30.0**	**3.4**	**10.6**	**7.1**	**6.9**	**ENGLAND AND WALES**
10.5	**28.0**	**3.3**	**10.0**	**6.9**	**6.2**	**England**
24.9	**66.8**	**6.5**	**21.5**	**11.4**	**19.4**	**Wales**
						Government Office Regions
16.4	26.8	*2.5*	26.8	17.9	*5.4*	North East
18.4	31.2	5.5	9.8	6.7	7.6	North West
5.9	22.3	*1.0*	7.1	5.1	3.5	Yorkshire and The Humber
18.8	57.7	*1.6*	18.3	13.4	8.5	East Midlands
6.5	18.7	*1.8*	3.5	*2.6*	4.7	West Midlands
6.8	18.1	3.9	8.7	7.0	6.8	East
6.4	19.1	4.7	7.1	4.5	5.8	London
6.9	22.0	*1.8*	10.1	7.0	6.2	South East
18.3	56.5	4.8	13.1	7.2	7.6	South West

Tables 6a and 6b 2004 Series MB3 no.19

Table 6a All babies notified - numbers:
month of birth by condition, 2004

Condition	Total	January	February	March	April	May	June
All babies notified	**6,358**	**581**	**587**	**579**	**569**	**547**	**543**
Babies with a mention of:							
Central nervous system anomalies	362	30	34	41	24	31	31
Anencephalus	22	1	1	4	1	1	3
All spina bifida	78	4	7	10	5	6	9
Eye	103	5	5	9	13	10	11
Cleft lip and palate	500	45	49	35	49	51	41
Other face, ear and neck	159	15	17	9	3	18	22
Heart and circulatory	1,234	121	105	113	121	96	129
Respiratory	146	22	13	17	12	12	13
Alimentary	416	41	32	31	35	35	32
Genital organs	521	42	47	56	40	35	48
Urinary system	725	59	82	64	72	70	55
Musculoskeletal	1,926	166	187	182	154	180	159
Skin and integument	220	22	21	15	19	20	24
Chromosomal anomalies	681	63	50	64	62	54	54
Down syndrome	456	43	28	39	43	32	36
Endocrine and metabolic disorders	153	15	15	15	16	11	10
Congenital infections	11	2	-	2	1	1	-
Other congenital anomalies not elsewhere classified	441	37	41	41	44	41	43
Total live and stillbirths	**643,026**	**53,351**	**49,620**	**53,048**	**51,660**	**52,985**	**53,603**

Table 6b All babies notified - rates per 10,000 total births:
month of birth by condition, 2004

Condition	Total	January	February	March	April	May	June
All babies notified	**98.9**	**108.9**	**118.3**	**109.1**	**110.1**	**103.2**	**101.3**
Babies with a mention of:							
Central nervous system anomalies	5.6	5.6	6.9	7.7	4.6	5.9	5.8
Anencephalus	0.3	0.2	0.2	0.8	0.2	0.2	0.6
All spina bifida	1.2	0.7	1.4	1.9	1.0	1.1	1.7
Eye	1.6	0.9	1.0	1.7	2.5	1.9	2.1
Cleft lip and palate	7.8	8.4	9.9	6.6	9.5	9.6	7.6
Other face, ear and neck	2.5	2.8	3.4	1.7	0.6	3.4	4.1
Heart and circulatory	19.2	22.7	21.2	21.3	23.4	18.1	24.1
Respiratory	2.3	4.1	2.6	3.2	2.3	2.3	2.4
Alimentary	6.5	7.7	6.4	5.8	6.8	6.6	6.0
Genital organs	8.1	7.9	9.5	10.6	7.7	6.6	9.0
Urinary system	11.3	11.1	16.5	12.1	13.9	13.2	10.3
Musculoskeletal	30.0	31.1	37.7	34.3	29.8	34.0	29.7
Skin and integument	3.4	4.1	4.2	2.8	3.7	3.8	4.5
Chromosomal anomalies	10.6	11.8	10.1	12.1	12.0	10.2	10.1
Down syndrome	7.1	8.1	5.6	7.4	8.3	6.0	6.7
Endocrine and metabolic disorders	2.4	2.8	3.0	2.8	3.1	2.1	1.9
Congenital infections	0.2	0.4	-	0.4	0.2	0.2	-
Other congenital anomalies not elsewhere classified	6.9	6.9	8.3	7.7	8.5	7.7	8.0

England and Wales

Month of birth						Condition
July	August	September	October	November	December	
534	**540**	**497**	**473**	**438**	**470**	**All babies notified**
						Babies with a mention of:
34	34	22	25	24	32	Central nervous system anomalies
1	3	1	3	2	1	Anencephalus
4	5	7	5	7	9	All spina bifida
13	3	6	11	10	7	Eye
46	44	30	42	32	36	Cleft lip and palate
12	12	9	19	9	14	Other face, ear and neck
90	102	104	97	85	71	Heart and circulatory
7	11	10	9	11	9	Respiratory
45	32	35	29	32	37	Alimentary
48	44	39	35	36	51	Genital organs
67	55	58	52	45	46	Urinary system
148	153	166	141	140	150	Musculoskeletal
18	28	10	12	14	17	Skin and integument
59	63	65	56	44	47	Chromosomal anomalies
40	40	46	44	34	31	Down syndrome
9	7	13	18	11	13	Endocrine and metabolic disorders
1	1	-	1	-	2	Congenital infections
33	34	29	38	24	36	Other congenital anomalies not elsewhere classified
55,927	**54,554**	**55,835**	**55,643**	**53,156**	**53,644**	**Total live and stillbirths**

England and Wales

Month of birth						Condition
July	August	September	October	November	December	
95.5	**99.0**	**89.0**	**85.0**	**82.4**	**87.6**	**All babies notified**
						Babies with a mention of:
6.1	6.2	3.9	4.5	4.5	6.0	Central nervous system anomalies
0.2	*0.5*	*0.2*	*0.5*	*0.4*	*0.2*	Anencephalus
0.7	*0.9*	*1.3*	*0.9*	*1.3*	*1.7*	All spina bifida
2.3	0.5	1.1	2.0	1.9	1.3	Eye
8.2	8.1	5.4	7.5	6.0	6.7	Cleft lip and palate
2.1	*2.2*	*1.6*	*3.4*	*1.7*	*2.6*	Other face, ear and neck
16.1	18.7	18.6	17.4	16.0	13.2	Heart and circulatory
1.3	*2.0*	*1.8*	*1.6*	*2.1*	*1.7*	Respiratory
8.0	5.9	6.3	5.2	6.0	6.9	Alimentary
8.6	8.1	7.0	6.3	6.8	9.5	Genital organs
12.0	10.1	10.4	9.3	8.5	8.6	Urinary system
26.5	28.0	29.7	25.3	26.3	28.0	Musculoskeletal
3.2	*5.1*	*1.8*	*2.2*	*2.6*	*3.2*	Skin and integument
10.5	11.5	11.6	10.1	8.3	8.8	Chromosomal anomalies
7.2	7.3	8.2	7.9	6.4	5.8	Down syndrome
1.6	*1.3*	*2.3*	*3.2*	*2.1*	*2.4*	Endocrine and metabolic disorders
0.2	*0.2*	-	*0.2*	-	*0.4*	Congenital infections
5.9	6.2	5.2	6.8	4.5	6.7	Other congenital anomalies not elsewhere classified

Table 7a 2004 Series MB3 no.19

Table 7a Live and stillborn babies notified - numbers: birthweight by condition, 2004 England and Wales

Condition			Birthweight (grammes)								
			Total[1]	Under 1,000	1,000-1,499	1,500-1,999	2,000-2,499	2,500-2,999	3,000-3,499	3,500 and over	Not stated
All babies notified	Total[2]	a	6,358	140	172	268	546	1,110	1,680	1,599	797
	Live born	b	6,023	59	137	234	511	1,094	1,656	1,586	725
	Stillborn	c	322	81	35	34	34	14	22	12	66
Babies with a mention of:											
Central nervous system anomalies		a	362	23	26	27	50	56	64	48	54
		b	277	7	17	17	38	53	60	47	33
		c	82	16	9	10	11	3	4	1	20
Anencephalus		a	22	4	3	4	1	2	1	-	4
		b	12	2	2	3	1	1	1	-	1
		c	10	2	1	1	-	1	-	-	3
All spina bifida		a	78	6	5	3	6	10	20	11	11
		b	58	1	3	3	5	10	20	11	4
		c	17	5	2	-	-	-	-	-	6
Eye		a	103	3	4	4	13	20	22	25	12
		b	99	2	4	3	12	20	21	25	12
		c	3	1	-	1	1	-	-	-	-
Cleft lip and palate		a	500	8	14	25	43	69	137	150	50
		b	483	5	12	22	41	69	136	150	46
		c	16	3	2	3	2	-	1	-	3
Other face, ear and neck		a	159	3	8	11	18	28	38	39	11
		b	151	3	7	8	18	28	37	39	9
		c	7	-	1	3	-	-	1	-	1
Heart and circulatory		a	1,234	39	35	60	109	219	251	228	282
		b	1,158	15	32	53	104	214	245	225	268
		c	74	24	3	7	5	4	6	3	13
Respiratory		a	146	8	10	14	10	27	28	26	20
		b	131	4	8	14	9	25	27	25	19
		c	15	4	2	-	1	2	1	1	1
Alimentary		a	416	14	18	30	56	82	96	78	41
		b	390	6	15	28	51	80	94	76	40
		c	25	8	3	2	5	1	2	2	1
Genital organs		a	521	9	15	20	38	88	163	157	29
		b	515	7	14	20	37	88	163	157	28
		c	6	2	1	-	1	-	-	-	1
Urinary system		a	725	10	18	27	55	119	204	216	71
		b	694	7	14	24	46	118	203	215	64
		c	29	3	4	3	9	1	1	1	5
Musculoskeletal		a	1,926	31	51	92	195	366	542	502	139
		b	1,855	14	45	82	186	362	537	501	126
		c	69	17	6	10	8	4	5	1	12
Skin and integument		a	220	1	3	7	8	44	69	74	12
		b	213	-	3	7	7	44	68	72	12
		c	5	1	-	-	1	-	-	1	-
Chromosomal anomalies		a	681	29	22	32	73	142	140	77	152
		b	596	6	15	25	66	138	133	75	130
		c	81	23	7	7	7	4	7	2	18
Down syndrome		a	456	11	11	15	50	112	117	49	87
		b	420	3	9	14	45	110	110	47	78
		c	34	8	2	1	5	2	7	2	7
Endocrine and metabolic disorders		a	153	4	4	9	17	31	35	39	14
		b	150	4	3	8	17	31	35	39	13
		c	3	-	1	1	-	-	-	-	1
Congenital infections		a	11	1	3	2	-	-	-	2	3
		b	9	-	3	2	-	-	-	2	2
		c	2	1	-	-	-	-	-	-	1
Other congenital anomalies not elsewhere classified		a	441	24	19	18	43	79	98	105	47
		b	382	8	7	14	38	78	93	103	38
		c	57	16	12	4	5	1	4	2	8
Total live and stillbirths		a	643,026	4,337	5,143	10,087	31,321	109,797	228,257	252,843	1,241
Live born		b	639,509	3,146	4,740	9,745	30,917	109,399	227,877	252,533	1,152
Stillborn		c	3,517	1,191	403	342	404	398	380	310	89

1 Total includes under 500 grammes although these are not included in the Under 1,000 column.
2 Total includes unknown whether live or stillborn.

Table 7b Live and stillborn babies notified - rates per 10,000 live/stillbirths: birthweight by condition, 2004

England and Wales

Condition			Birthweight (grammes)								
			Total[1]	Under 1,000	1,000-1,499	1,500-1,999	2,000-2,499	2,500-2,999	3,000-3,499	3,500 and over	Not stated
All babies notified	Live born	a	94.2	187.5	289.0	240.1	165.3	100.0	72.7	62.8	6,293.4
	Stillborn	b	915.6	680.1	868.5	994.2	841.6	351.8	578.9	387.1	7,415.7
Babies with a mention of:											
Central nervous system anomalies		a	4.3	22.3	35.9	17.4	12.3	4.8	2.6	1.9	286.5
		b	233.2	134.3	223.3	292.4	272.3	75.4	105.3	32.3	2,247.2
Anencephalus		a	0.2	6.4	4.2	3.1	0.3	0.1	0.0	-	8.7
		b	28.4	16.8	24.8	29.2	-	25.1	-	-	337.1
All spina bifida		a	0.9	3.2	6.3	3.1	1.6	0.9	0.9	0.4	34.7
		b	48.3	42.0	49.6	-	-	-	-	-	674.2
Eye		a	1.5	6.4	8.4	3.1	3.9	1.8	0.9	1.0	104.2
		b	8.5	8.4	-	29.2	24.8	-	-	-	-
Cleft lip and palate		a	7.6	15.9	25.3	22.6	13.3	6.3	6.0	5.9	399.3
		b	45.5	25.2	49.6	87.7	49.5	-	26.3	-	337.1
Other face, ear and neck		a	2.4	9.5	14.8	8.2	5.8	2.6	1.6	1.5	78.1
		b	19.9	-	24.8	87.7	-	-	26.3	-	112.4
Heart and circulatory		a	18.1	47.7	67.5	54.4	33.6	19.6	10.8	8.9	2,326.4
		b	210.4	201.5	74.4	204.7	123.8	100.5	157.9	96.8	1,460.7
Respiratory		a	2.0	12.7	16.9	14.4	2.9	2.3	1.2	1.0	164.9
		b	42.7	33.6	49.6	-	24.8	50.3	26.3	32.3	112.4
Alimentary		a	6.1	19.1	31.6	28.7	16.5	7.3	4.1	3.0	347.2
		b	71.1	67.2	74.4	58.5	123.8	25.1	52.6	64.5	112.4
Genital organs		a	8.1	22.3	29.5	20.5	12.0	8.0	7.2	6.2	243.1
		b	17.1	16.8	24.8	-	24.8	-	-	-	112.4
Urinary system		a	10.9	22.3	29.5	24.6	14.9	10.8	8.9	8.5	555.6
		b	82.5	25.2	99.3	87.7	222.8	25.1	26.3	32.3	561.8
Musculoskeletal		a	29.0	44.5	94.9	84.1	60.2	33.1	23.6	19.8	1,093.8
		b	196.2	142.7	148.9	292.4	198.0	100.5	131.6	32.3	1,348.3
Skin and integument		a	3.3	-	6.3	7.2	2.3	4.0	3.0	2.9	104.2
		b	14.2	8.4	-	-	24.8	-	-	32.3	-
Chromosomal anomalies		a	9.3	19.1	31.6	25.7	21.3	12.6	5.8	3.0	1,128.5
		b	230.3	193.1	173.7	204.7	173.3	100.5	184.2	64.5	2,022.5
Down syndrome		a	6.6	9.5	19.0	14.4	14.6	10.1	4.8	1.9	677.1
		b	96.7	67.2	49.6	29.2	123.8	50.3	184.2	64.5	786.5
Endocrine and metabolic disorders		a	2.3	12.7	6.3	8.2	5.5	2.8	1.5	1.5	112.8
		b	8.5	-	24.8	29.2	-	-	-	-	112.4
Congenital infections		a	0.1	-	6.3	2.1	-	-	-	0.1	17.4
		b	5.7	8.4	-	-	-	-	-	-	112.4
Other congenital anomalies not elsewhere classified		a	6.0	25.4	14.8	14.4	12.3	7.1	4.1	4.1	329.9
		b	162.1	134.3	297.8	117.0	123.8	25.1	105.3	64.5	898.9

1 Total includes under 500 grammes although these are not included in the Under 1,000 column

Table 8a All babies notified - numbers: age of mother by condition, 2004

England and Wales

Condition	Total[1]	Under 20	20-24	25-29	30-34	35-39	40-44	45 and over
All babies notified	6,358	558	1,212	1,449	1,621	1,027	268	15
Babies with a mention of:								
Central nervous system anomalies	362	40	74	78	91	55	17	1
Anencephalus	22	3	6	5	3	4	-	-
All spina bifida	78	10	12	16	23	10	7	-
Eye	103	6	19	19	26	23	6	-
Cleft lip and palate	500	45	87	116	148	67	17	1
Other face, ear and neck	159	9	28	41	41	22	12	-
Heart and circulatory	1,234	104	224	270	293	204	59	5
Respiratory	146	17	33	24	46	19	3	-
Alimentary	416	39	70	91	102	83	14	2
Genital organs	521	50	92	139	136	77	21	1
Urinary system	725	58	160	159	208	113	20	1
Musculoskeletal	1,926	215	410	466	477	272	59	1
Skin and integument	220	11	43	58	61	29	13	-
Chromosomal anomalies	681	29	58	90	163	186	97	10
Down syndrome	456	16	35	54	101	145	70	3
Endocrine and metabolic disorders	153	11	36	34	31	23	8	-
Congenital infections	11	2	5	3	1	-	-	-
Other congenital anomalies not elsewhere classified	441	30	96	106	113	74	13	1
Total live and stillbirths	643,026	45,415	121,731	160,751	191,402	102,760	20,049	918

1 Totals include age not stated

Table 8b All babies notified - rates per 10,000 total births: age of mother by condition, 2004

England and Wales

Condition	Total[1]	Under 20	20-24	25-29	30-34	35-39	40-44	45 and over
All babies notified	98.9	122.9	99.6	90.1	84.7	99.9	133.7	*163.4*
Babies with a mention of:								
Central nervous system anomalies	5.6	8.8	6.1	4.9	4.8	5.4	8.5	*10.9*
Anencephalus	0.3	*0.7*	*0.5*	*0.3*	*0.2*	*0.4*	-	-
All spina bifida	1.2	2.2	*1.0*	*1.0*	1.2	*1.0*	*3.5*	-
Eye	1.6	*1.3*	*1.6*	*1.2*	1.4	2.2	*3.0*	-
Cleft lip and palate	7.8	9.9	7.1	7.2	7.7	6.5	8.5	*10.9*
Other face, ear and neck	2.5	2.0	2.3	2.6	2.1	2.1	*6.0*	-
Heart and circulatory	19.2	22.9	18.4	16.8	15.3	19.9	29.4	*54.5*
Respiratory	2.3	*3.7*	2.7	1.5	2.4	*1.8*	*1.5*	-
Alimentary	6.5	8.6	5.8	5.7	5.3	8.1	*7.0*	*21.8*
Genital organs	8.1	*11.0*	7.6	8.6	7.1	7.5	*10.5*	*10.9*
Urinary system	11.3	12.8	13.1	9.9	10.9	11.0	10.0	*10.9*
Musculoskeletal	30.0	47.3	33.7	29.0	24.9	26.5	29.4	*10.9*
Skin and integument	3.4	*2.4*	3.5	3.6	3.2	2.8	*6.5*	-
Chromosomal anomalies	10.6	6.4	4.8	5.6	8.5	18.1	48.4	*108.9*
Down syndrome	7.1	*3.5*	2.9	3.4	5.3	14.1	34.9	*32.7*
Endocrine and metabolic disorders	2.4	*2.4*	3.0	2.1	1.6	2.2	*4.0*	-
Congenital infections	*0.2*	*0.4*	*0.4*	*0.2*	*0.1*	-	-	-
Other congenital anomalies not elsewhere classified	6.9	6.6	7.9	6.6	5.9	7.2	*6.5*	*10.9*

1 Totals include age not stated

Table 9 Strategic Health Authorities in England, and Wales which have shown an increase of numbers of a particular anomaly compared with the average notification for that area and anomaly during a previous period, 2004

ONS Monitoring group[1]	Anomaly	Strategic Health Authority	Quarter
0E	Encephalocele	Leicestershire, Northamptonshire and Rutland	June
C	**Alimentary System**	South Yorkshire	September
2C	Cleft palate with cleft lip	Cumbria and Lancashire	December
2E	Atresia/stenosis of large intestine, rectum & anal canal	Bedfordshire and Hertfordshire	June
D	**Cardiovascular System**	North Central London South West London South Yorkshire Wales	March March June December
3A	Tetralogy of Fallot	South West London	June
3B	Ventricular septal defect	Greater Manchester Avon, Gloucestershire and Wiltshire Shropshire and Staffordshire Wales	June March December December
3C	Other septal defects	South Yorkshire Wales	June December
3E	Patent ductus arteriosus	North West London Avon, Gloucestershire and Wiltshire South West Peninsula South Yorkshire	December June June March
3F	Anomalies of the umbilical artery	Avon, Gloucestershire and Wiltshire	September
3G	Other congenital cardiac or great vessel anomalies	Wales	December
3H	Congenital anomalies of other vessels	South Yorkshire	June, September
E	**Respiratory System**	Bedfordshire and Hertfordshire Dorset and Somerset	March December
5J	Congenital obstructive defects of renal pelvis or anomalies of ureter	Avon, Gloucestershire and Wiltshire Birmingham and the Black Country	June March, September
G	**Limbs**	South West Peninsula	September, December
6D	Dislocation of hip	Avon, Gloucestershire and Wiltshire	March, September
H	**Other Musculoskeletal**	Avon, Gloucestershire and Wiltshire South West Peninsula	September March
7D	Osteodystrophy or chondrodystrophy	Northumberland, Tyne & Wear Birmingham and the Black Country	June March
7G	Exomphalos	North East London	March
7H	Anomalies of the lips, tongue and pharynx	Cumbria and Lancashire	December
7K	Congenital diaphragmatic hernia	Hampshire and Isle of Wight	December
7L	Gastroschisis	Northumberland, Tyne & Wear Thames Valley Wales	December June June
7P	Other anomalies of face & neck	Thames Valley	June, September
I	**Skin and Integument**	Norfolk, Suffolk and Cambridgeshire North East London South East London Cumbria and Lancashire	March June June, December September
9C	Trisomy 21 - Down syndrome	County Durham and Tees Valley Leicestershire, Northamptonshire and Rutland	June September
9D	Other chromosomal anomalies	Avon, Gloucestershire and Wiltshire Wales	March March

1 See Appendix D

Appendix A - List of conditions for exclusion

Reports of cases with the following anomalies are not to be transmitted to ONS unless occurring in combination with other anomalies:

Name of condition

Spina bifida occulta uncomplicated
Stenosis or stricture of lacrimal duct
Minor or unspecified anomaly of auricle
Minor or unspecified anomaly of nose
Minor or unspecified deformity of face
Minor anomaly of nipple, accessory or ectopic nipple
Congenital umbilical hernia, inguinal or para umbilical
Undescended testicle and unspecified ectopic testis
Congenital hydrocele or hydrocele of testis
Phimosis
Hypospadias when the meatus lies before the coronary sulcus
Abnormal palmar crease
Skin tag with surface less than 4 cm^2: skin tag, naevus, angioma, haemangioma, glomus tumour, lymphangioma, birthmark
Clicking hip
Clubfoot of postural original
Minor or unspecified anomalies of toe such as hallux valgus, hallux varus or "orteuil en marteau"
Functional or unspecified cardiac murmur
Absence or hypoplasia of umbilical artery, single umbilical artery

With acknowledgement to EUROCAT for permission to reproduce their exclusion list.

Appendix B - Example of congenital anomaly form (SD56)

CONGENITAL ANOMALIES — Form SD56

Identification number: ....
(The form of this number is not important, but should be decided locally to enable a particular case to be identified subsequently if required.)

NHS number of child: ☐☐☐☐☐☐☐☐☐☐

Health Authority of mother's usual residence: .... HA

Health Authority in which baby was born: → .... HA

Surname of child (first three characters only): → ☐☐☐

Forename of child (first three characters only): → ☐☐☐

Place of birth of child (please tick one box only): → Home ☐₁ NHS Hospital ☐₂ Other ☐₃ Not known ☐

If 'Other', please specify ....

Date of birth of child: → (day) ☐☐ (month) ☐☐ (year) ☐☐☐☐

Sex of child (please tick one box only): → Male ☐₁ Female ☐₂ Indeterminate ☐₃ Not known ☐

Whether live or still birth (please tick one box only): → Live ☐₁ Born live, died within 7 days ☐₂ Stillborn ☐₃

Whether single or multiple birth (please enter number): → Single ☐ If multiple, state number born ☐

Date of LMP: → (day) ☐☐ (month) ☐☐ (year) ☐☐☐☐

If LMP date not known, state estimated gestation: → ☐☐ weeks

Birthweight: → ☐☐☐☐ grammes

Home address of mother: ....
....
....

(Please include postcode if known) → Postcode ☐☐☐☐☐☐☐

Parents' occupation (just before or early in mother's pregnancy):

Mother: ....

Father: ....

Date of birth of mother: → (day) ☐☐ (month) ☐☐ (year) ☐☐☐☐

If date of birth not known, state age: → ☐☐ years

Number and outcome of previous pregnancies resulting in: → Live births ☐ Stillbirths ☐ Others* ☐

Status of informant (please tick one box only): → Doctor ☐₁ Midwife ☐₂ Other ☐₃

If 'Other', please specify ....

Congenital anomalies reported:

(A detailed written description of each congenital anomaly is needed so that ONS can code the anomalies to the 4-digit ICD classification. **It is important that no anomalies are omitted.**)

....
....
....
....
....
....
....

---

* 'Others' is defined as pregnancies that ended in other than a registrable live or stillbirth.

TA15/3 12/98

Appendix C - List of ICD10 codes included within anomaly groups

Anomaly Group	Congenital Anomaly description	ICD10 codes used for data on the National Congenital Anomaly System	ICD10 codes used in Table 1 and Appendix E (Abortions, Stillbirths and Neonatal deaths)
Central nervous system	All	G04.9, G12.0, G12.9, G40.9, G60.0, G62.9, G70.9, G71.1, G71.2, G80.9, G83.2, G93.0, G93.1, Q00-Q07	Q00-Q07
	Anencephalus	Q00	Q00
	All spina bifida	Q05	Q05
	Encephalocele	Q01	Q01
	Congenital hydrocephalus	Q03	Q03
Eye	All	H18.5, H50.0, H50.8, H54.0, H54.4, H55, Q10-Q15	Q10-Q15
	Anophthalmia	Q11.0-Q11.2	Q11.0-Q11.2
Cleft lip and palate	All	Q35-Q37	Q35-Q37
	Cleft of lip only	Q36	Q36
	Cleft of palate only	Q35	Q35
	Cleft of lip and palate	Q37	Q37
Other face, ear and neck	All	K07, Q16-Q18, R22.0, R22.1	Q16-Q18
Heart and circulatory	All	I45.6, I47.1, I49.1, M30.3, Q20-Q28	Q20-Q28
Respiratory	All	Q30-Q34	Q30-Q34
Alimentary	All	K74.0, K80.2, Q38-Q45, R14	Q38-Q45
	Tracheo-oesophageal fistula	Q39.1-Q39.3	Q39.1-Q39.3
	Oesophageal atresia	Q39.0	Q39.0
	Atresia/stenosis large intestine, rectum or anal canal	Q42	Q42
Genital organs	All	N47, N89.8, Q50-Q56	Q50-Q56
	Hypospadias	Q54	Q54
Urinary system	All	N13.9, N25.8, Q60-Q64	Q60-Q64
	Renal agenesis/dysgenesis	Q60	Q60
	Epispadias	Q64.0	Q64.0
Musculoskeletal	All	K40-K46, M21.2, M89.8, P94, Q65-Q79	Q65-Q79
	Dislocation of the hip	Q65.0-Q65.6	Q65.0-Q65.6
	Deformities of feet	Q66	Q66
	Polydactyly	Q69	Q69
	Syndactyly	Q70	Q70
	Limb reductions	Q71-Q73	Q71-Q73
	Diaphragmatic defects	Q79.0-Q79.1	Q79.0-Q79.1
	Exomphalos	Q79.2	Q79.2
	Gastroschisis	Q79.3	Q79.3
Skin and integument	All	D18.0, D22.3, D22.6, D22.7, D22.9, D23.6, D23.7, L53.9, L81.3, Q80-Q84	Q80-Q84
Chromosomal anomalies	All	Q90-Q99	Q90-Q99
	Down syndrome	Q90	Q90
Endocrine and metabolic disorders	All	D66, D67, D68.0, D68.2, D69.4, D81.9, D82.1, E03.0, E03.1, E07, E23-E25, E27-E30, E32, E34, E70-E80, E83-E85, E88, E90	
Congenital infections	All	A50.0, P29.4, P35, P37, P52.5	
Other anomalies not elsewhere classified	All	B27.0, C49.2, C69.2, C71.9, C74.9, D13.9, D14.3, D15.1, D16.6, D17.2, D17.9, D18.1, D36.1, D37.0, D41.0, D43.2, D47.1, D48.0, D48.7, D48.9, D55.0, D56.3, D57.1, D57.3, D58.0, F79, I42.4, K21.9, L05.9, P02.6, P10-P15, P20-P29, (excl P29.4), P36, P50, P61, P70-P78, P80-P83, P90-P93, P95, P96, Q85-Q89, R16.0, R16.2, R18, R19.0, R22.9	Q85-Q89

Appendix D - ONS Monitoring groups and ICD10 equivalent codes

		ICD10 Codes
Central Nervous System	**A**	
0A	Anencephalus	Q00.0-Q00.2
0B	Spina bifida	Q05.0-Q05.9
0C	Congenital hydrocephalus	Q03.0-Q03.9
0E	Encephalocele	Q01.0-Q01.9
0F	Other	G04.9, G12.0, G12.9, G40.9, G60.0, G62.9, G70.9, G71.1, G71.2, G80.9, G83.2, G93.0, G93.1, Q02, Q04, Q06, Q07
Eye and Ear	**B**	
1A	Cystic eyeball	Q11.0
1B	Congenital lens anomalies	Q12.0-Q12.9
1C	Other & unspecified eye anomalies	Q10, Q11.3, Q13-Q15, H18.5, H 50.0, H50.8, H54.0, H54.4, H55
1D	Ear, all	Q16, Q17
1E	Other anophthalmos	Q11.1-Q11.2
Alimentary System	**C**	
2A	Cleft of palate only	Q35
2B	Cleft of lip only	Q36
2C	Cleft palate with cleft lip	Q37
2D	Tracheo-oesophageal fistula/stenosis	Q39.0-Q39.3
2E	Atresia/stenosis of large intestine, rectum & anal canal	Q42.0-Q42.9
2F	Other or unspecified anomalies of alimentary system	K74.0, K80.2, Q39.4-Q39.9, Q40.0, Q40.2-Q40.9, Q41, Q43-Q45, R14
Cardiovascular System	**D**	
3A	Tetralogy of Fallot	Q21.3
3B	Ventricular septal defect	Q21.0
3C	Other septal defects	Q21.1-Q21.2, Q21.4-Q21.9
3E	Patent ductus arteriosus	Q25.0
3F	Anomalies of the umbilical artery	Q27.0
3G	Other congenital cardiac or great vessel anomalies	I45.6, I47.1, I49.1, M30.3, Q20, Q22-Q24, Q25.1-Q25.9, Q26
3H	Congenital anomalies of other vessels	Q27.1-Q27.9, Q28
Respiratory System	**E**	
4A	Congenital anomalies of the respiratory system	Q30-Q34
Urogenital System	**F**	
5A	Hypospadias/epispadias	Q54, Q64.0
5B	Other anomalies of the male genitalia	N47, Q53, Q55
5C	Anomalies of the female genitalia	N89.8, Q50-Q52
5D	Bladder exstrophy	Q64.1
5E	Renal agenesis	Q60
5F	Other or unspecified defects of urogenital system	N25.8, Q63, Q64.2-Q64.9
5G	Indeterminate sex	Q56
5H	Cystic kidney disease	Q61
5J	Congenital obstructive defects of renal pelvis or anomalies of ureter	N13.9, Q62
Limbs	**G**	
6A	Polydactyly/syndactyly	Q69, Q70
6B	Limb reductions	Q71-Q73
6C	Deformities of feet	Q66
6D	Dislocation of hip	Q65.0-Q65.6
6E	Other limb or limb girdles	M21.2, Q65.8, Q65.9, Q68.1-Q68.5, Q74
Other Musculoskeletal	**H**	
7A	Other anomalies of the diaphragm	Q79.1
7B	Anomalies of the face, skull or neck	Q67-Q68.0, Q75, R22.0
7C	Other musculoskeletal anomalies of the thorax and neck	Q76.8, Q76.9
7D	Osteodystrophy or chondrodystrophy	Q77, Q78
7E	Other or unspecified anomalies of the musculoskeletal system	M89.8, P94, Q68.8, Q76.0-Q76.7, Q79.5, Q79.9
7F	Anomalies of the abdominal wall (hernias)	K40-K46
7G	Exomphalos	Q79.2
7H	Anomalies of the lips, tongue and pharynx	Q18.4-Q18.7, Q38
7J	Congenital hiatus hernia	Q40.1
7K	Congenital diaphragmatic hernia	Q79.0
7L	Gastroschisis	Q79.3
7M	Prune belly syndrome	Q79.4
7N	Branchial cleft, auricular sinus	Q18.0-Q18.2
7P	Other anomalies of face & neck	K07, Q18.3, Q18.8, Q18.9, R22.1

Skin and Integument   **I**
8C   Anomalies of the skin or integument   D18.0, D22.3, D22.6, D22.7, D22.9, D23.6, D23.7, L53.9, L81.3, Q80-Q84

Other Anomalies   **K**
9A   Congenital neoplasms (other than benign skin)   C49.2, C69.2, C71.9, C74.9, D13.9, D14.3, D15.1, D16.6, D17.2, D17.9, D36.1, D37.0, D41.0, D43.2, D47.1, D48.0, D48.7, D48.9

9B   Endocrine and metabolic disorders   D66, D67, D68.0, D68.2, D69.4, D81.9, D82.1, E03.0, E03.1, E07, E23-E25, E27-E30, E32, E34, E70-E80, E83-E85, E88, E90

9C   Trisomy 21 - Down syndrome   Q90
9D   Other chromosomal anomalies   Q91-Q99
9E   Other and unspecified congenital anomalies   B27.0, D18.1, D55.0, D56.3, D57.1, D57.3, D58.0, F79, I42.4, K21.9, L05.9, P02.6, P10-P15, P20-P29 (excl P29.4), P36, P50, P61, P70-P78, P80-P83, P90-P93, P95, P96, Q85-Q89, R16.0, R16.2, R18, R19.0, R22.9

9H   Congenital infections   A50.0, P29.4, P35, P37, P52.5

**Appendix E Summary table showing congenital anomaly statistics from three systems
National Congenital Anomaly System, Abortion Statistics, Mortality Statistics, 2003**

England and Wales

Condition	Congenital anomaly notifications (NCAS)[1]			Abortion notifications (under grounds E)[2]	Stillbirths - occurrences with a fetal mention[3]		Neonatal deaths- occurrences with a fetal mention[3]	
	Live birth	Stillbirth	Not known		Main	Other	Main	Other
All babies notified	6,624	332	27	1,941	437	247	432	387
Babies with a mention of:								
Central nervous system anomalies	260	95	1	486	105	44	63	35
Anencephalus	17	16	-	159	21	2	23	1
All spina bifida	57	23	1	118	22	7	4	4
Encephalocele	9	-	-	20	1	-	2	4
Congenital hydrocephalus	56	17	-	55	29	9	13	2
Eye	88	1	1	*	-	-	1	1
Anophthalmia	10	-	-	*	-	-	-	-
Cleft lip and palate	509	15	2	*	2	5	3	5
Cleft of only lip	130	2	-	*	-	2	-	-
Cleft of only palate	170	5	1	*	1	-	1	3
Cleft of lip and palate	209	8	1	*	1	3	2	2
Other face, ear and neck	226	9	-	*	3	2	2	-
Heart and circulatory	1,261	56	5	108	87	70	143	115
Respiratory	133	17	-	25	4	5	61	34
Alimentary	414	14	-	*	11	6	7	22
Tracheo-oesophageal fistula	47	-	-	*	1	-	2	5
Oesophageal atresia	13	1	-	*	1	-	1	4
Atresia/stenosis large intestine, rectum or anal canal	79	3	-	*	-	-	1	2
Genital organs	592	9	4	*	-	-	-	3
Hypospadias	456	1	1	*	-	-	-	1
Urinary system	745	35	3	78	33	16	33	43
Renal agenesis/dysgenesis	69	10	1	26	12	1	12	15
Epispadias	13	-	-	*	-	-	-	-
Musculoskeletal	1,922	84	10	120	46	41	51	60
Dislocation of hip	107	-	-	*	-	-	-	-
Deformities of feet	601	18	3	*	3	8	2	-
Polydactyly	350	6	-	*	-	1	-	-
Syndactyly	221	6	1	*	-	-	-	-
Limb reductions	171	18	2	11	1	4	-	1
Diaphragmatic defects	75	8	1	16	4	3	24	20
Exomphalos	48	7	-	*	8	5	2	10
Gastroschisis	129	2	1	*	4	2	2	3
Skin and integument	270	1	-	*	-	-	1	2
Chromosomal anomalies	521	75	-	709	78	28	46	26
Down syndrome	350	24	-	401	22	12	6	12
Endocrine and metabolic disorders	171	7	-	*	-	-	-	-
Congenital infections	12	5	-	..	-	-	-	-
Other congenital anomalies not elsewhere classified	554	60	4	85	68	30	21	40

Source
1 National Congenital Anomaly System at 4th November 2004.
2 Department of Health. Abortion Statistics, England and Wales 2003, July 2005.
3 Office for National Statistics. Series DH3 no. 36, Mortality Statistics: Childhood, infant and perinatal, 2003.

* less than 10 cases